Diet Programs and your Health

Knowing More about Proper and Healthy Diet Programs

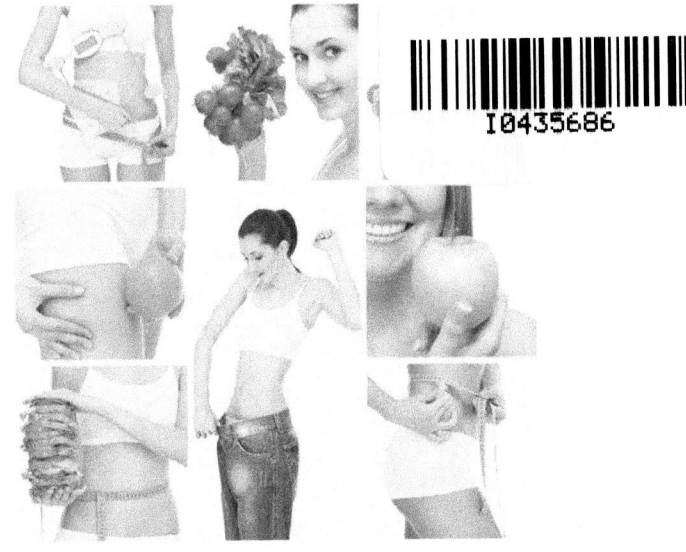

I0435686

Natural Health Series

Dueep J Singh

Mendon Cottage Books

JD-Biz Publishing

Disclaimer

The information is this book is provided for informational purposes only. It is not intended to be used and medical advice or a substitute for proper medical treatment by a qualified health care provider. The information is believed to be accurate as presented based on research by the author.

The contents have not been evaluated by the U.S. Food and Drug Administration or any other Government or Health Organization and the contents in this book are not to be used to treat cure or prevent disease.

The author or publisher is not responsible for the use or safety of any diet, procedure or treatment mentioned in this book. The author or publisher is not responsible for errors or omissions that may exist.

Warning

The Book is for informational purposes only and before taking on any diet, treatment or medical procedure, it is recommended to consult with your primary health care provider.

Check out some of the other Healthy Gardening Series books at Amazon.com

Gardening Series on Amazon

Check out some of the other Health Learning Series books at Amazon.com

Health Learning Series on Amazon

Table of Contents

Introduction

Did you know that the concept of dieting is a relatively modern one? In ancient times, the mere idea of going without food, in order to lose weight was not very common or usual. That is because most of the time, a large majority of people did not have enough of food to eat. So the idea of their becoming fat was reduced.

Also, our ancestors made sure that they spent a major part of their lives doing hard physical labor in the open air. That is why the food that they ate was easily assimilated in their bodies. This meant that there was no chance of their gaining extra weight or the accumulation of extra cellulite on any part of their bodies.

Man was naturally conditioned through his genes to have a protective layer of fat on his body. That is why down the centuries, the idea of no fat on a body did not disturb his equanimity. You may want to look at all the paintings and statues down the centuries. The women and even children are Ruben-esque in nature, which means they are chubby and plump.

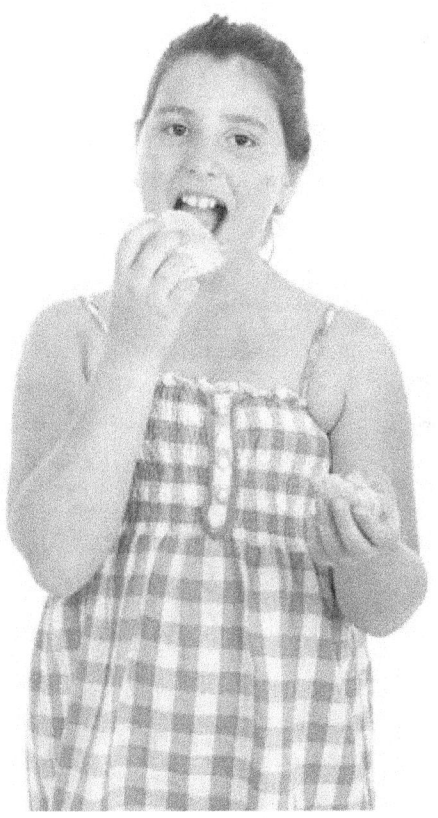

Bad eating habits inculcated in childhood means unhealthy adults.

That shows that in those days, the idea of beauty was a well fed, well-rounded human being. It showed that that person belonged to a family, which could afford to feed the children and the other adult members of the family so well that they would afford to grow fat!

This condition continued to the late 19th century, when better industrial conditions began to improve the standard of living. The production of more and more food meant that eating habits changed. People could afford to grow fat, because they had access to more food.

And so the idea of dieting started as a fad, especially in Europe, where the concept of slimness began to be considered to be synonymous with youth and everlasting beauty.

It was only after the First World War that the concept of slim is beautiful, began to insinuate itself into the social concept of beauty. Being thin as a stick began to be looked on as attractive.

That was because during the First World War, thanks to the paucity of food, most of the populace was starving so the idea of fashion designers designing clothes for "fat" people was not practical.

That is where the androgynous look came into the annals of fashion, with skinny, Twiggy, anorexic and skeletal bodies being considered to be beautiful, especially in women. Even so, the very thin females and males were not called slim, they were called skinny. And the mental aspiration of ideal measurements of 40 – 24 – 36, for a "womanly" figure still persists to this day.

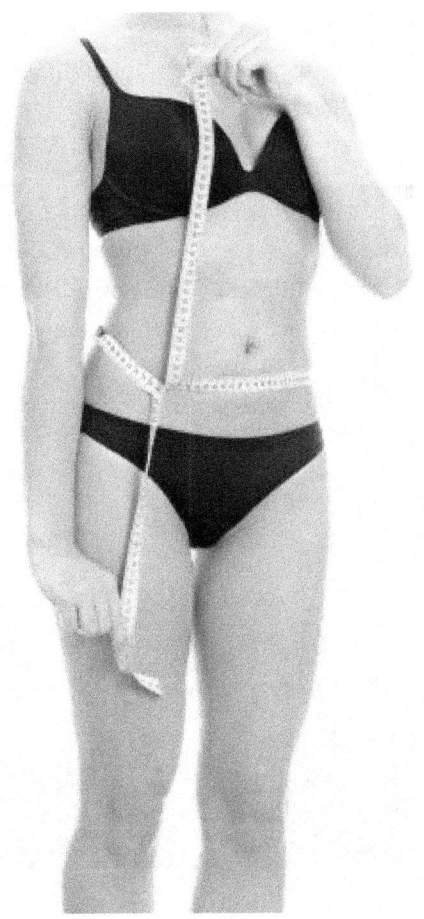

Getting obsessed with losing weight or your measurements is not very healthy, especially when you begin measuring yourself or weighing yourself after every meal.

Difference between Dieting and Fasting

For centuries people have been going on "fasts" for different reasons. In ancient times, fasting was done for the purification of body and soul. You can consider this to be a detoxification method in which one abstains totally from taking any kind of food. This is a totally voluntary activity which you are doing of your own will.

It is definitely different from starvation, which happens when you do not have access to food. That means you are not getting enough of food which your body needs. Your body is now going to suffer from malnutrition, because it is being starved.

In ancient times, people who went on a fast did not take any sort of solid, liquid food, cereals, fruit, vegetables and some people also did not drink any water. This sort of strict fasting has come down the ages, especially as a religious tradition to purify heart, body, mind, soul and spirit.

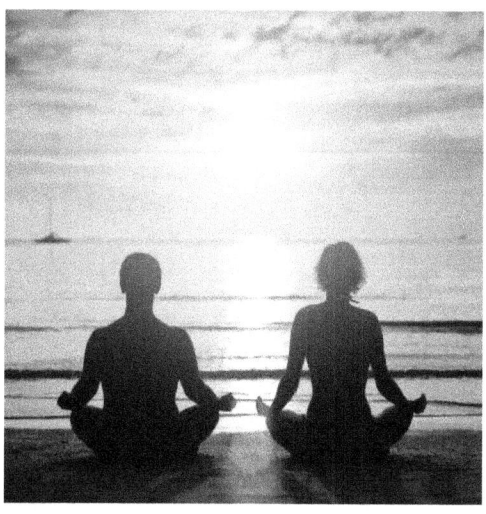

For many people down the ages, fasting was a religious ritual, along with meditation and prayers.

This food is not taken for a definite period of time, and for a definite purpose. On the other hand, dieting means that you are not going to be taking some particular items of food.

You however are going to be taking some sort of sustenance in some form or the other. This is going to include fruit, liquids and other requisite food items, required by your body to keep healthy. These include cereals, and other natural food items which are going to keep your body replenished with vitamins, minerals, carbohydrates, proteins, and other food-based nutrients.

Consider a diet to be some sort of "fasting" when you are not going to totally abstain from taking food. Remember that the more food you eat, the chances of toxins accumulating in your body are going to increase proportionately. Total abstinence from taking any sort of food and water is going to get rid of all these toxins.

But as this is not a healthy alternative – because it means that your body is starving itself thanks to the lack of proper nutrients needed to keep it functioning properly – the other alternative is a strict diet regime.

People generally believe that the existence and basis of strength in your body is dependent in on your food intake. They have the feeling that if they miss a meal, they are going to feel weak. In some ways, this is true, because that means your body is exhausted, and it does not have an immediate fuel source with which to replenish itself.

However, that is not what the ancients believed. According to them regular fastings kept them healthy, rejuvenated and energetic.

But as we do not intend to starve ourselves by depriving our bodies of nutritious meals, regularly and around 3 times a day, we need to have regulated diets which are going to help us keep healthy and happy.

You may ask me if I know anybody who has benefited through fasting. Well, I can say yes, an aunt of mine [1] who suffered from cancer and was clinically declared dead *twice* by her doctors in France, suddenly decided that she had had enough of expensive chemotherapy and drugs. So she decided to come back home and cure herself naturally.

She stopped eating everything solid [read "cooked"] and lived on for the next 25 years on just fruit and vegetables from her garden and fruit juice. Absolutely nothing else. And as this is the diet which was normally followed by ancients of long ago, it is possible that that kept her healthy and alive all these years.

Now, I consider this to be a great display of willpower. But this shows that there are some people who survive on such a diet. I do not have that willpower or the dedication to do so. Besides, my aunt had a spiritual bent

---

[1] The Late Brinder Aulakh - Tarot Card Reader, linguist, author and educationist - (d- Sept.2012)

of mind, and could resist the lure of delicious gourmet meals! I could not and do not. So that is why, I write so extensively on healthy diets and nutritive foods.

Low Carbohydrate Cooking

The obsession with weight gain and weight loss is getting to be more all-pervasive, all over the world and that is the reason why so many people are suffering from eating disorders. They do not want to accept the fact that they are suffering from starvation and malnutrition. According to them, they are dieting to lose weight because it is so not cool to be fat.

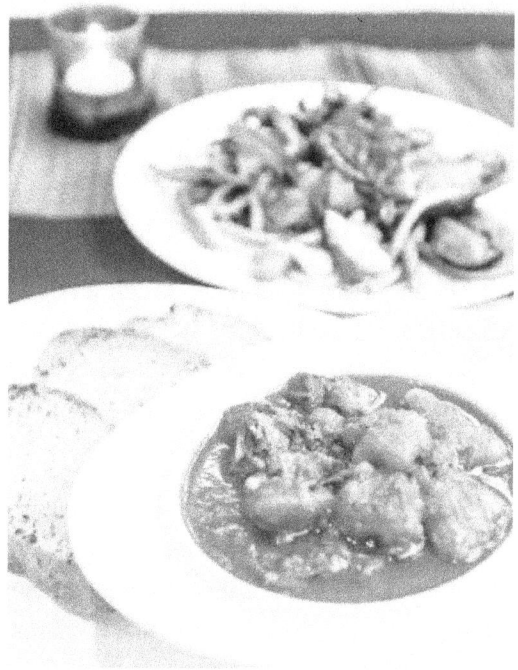

The meat may look rich, and full of butter, but it is high on protein and low on carbohydrates. And if the bread is made of soybean, it is a good meal combination.

Fashion dictates say that we have to be as thin as rakes. Many times health problems also say that we need to control our lives in order to keep healthy and keep alive.

That is why we go on drastic diets, starving our bodies of the essential nutrients, minerals, proteins and carbohydrates necessary to keep it working properly. There are so many diet programs in the market, being touted about by people As the Absolutely Last Thing in Weight Loss.

These include the Mayo Clinic diet – which incidentally has nothing to do with the Mayo Clinic, – you are going to take hard cooked eggs for about 10 days. This is a terribly harmful diet, because you are depriving your body of necessary and essential nutrition. Follow the diet and you are on your way to starvation.

Calorie Counting Diets

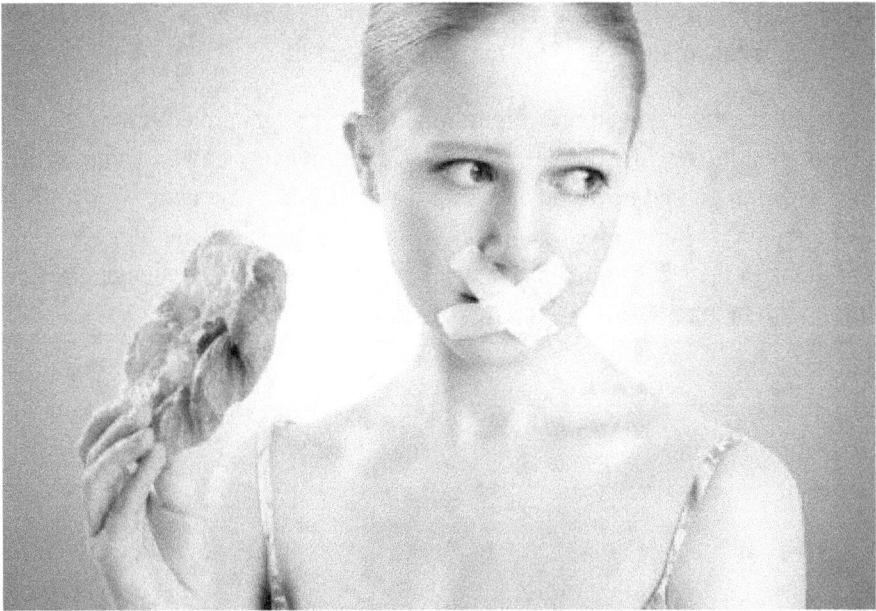

I was astonished to see a healthy 10-year-old girl making a diet chart of the calories taken in her meals, and weighing herself morning and night. When I asked her why she was doing so, she told me that her mother had told her that she was fat. Now, I have not come across a more blatant example of parental stupidity.

Not only is the mother causing her child to feel low self-esteem, but she has already set her on the way to future eating disorders.

Bulimia and anorexia are just harmful side effects of calorie counting diets. A 10-year-old child has absolutely no business counting calories, especially when she is a healthy child. Also, the idea of weighing herself morning and night is something psychologically abnormal.

But I knew the mother. She was obsessed with weight loss and weight gain. She was the first one to try out any diet, in the market and spent her paycheck on the latest weight-loss fad being followed by the stars. She was ruining her health steadily in an almost neurotic manner. And any diet that she followed had to be followed by the rest of the family, or else pandemonium in the house .

So now, thanks to her, her child had begun to obsess about weight loss and weight gain, at a very young age, when she should have been eating healthy nutritive meals in order to grow into a healthy adult.

Remember, obsessing about weight loss and weight gain to extremes is definitely not a healthy mental outlook. Counting every calorie eaten, and then worrying about how you are going to get it off, is one way, why so many people suffer from stress, tension and other physical and mental problems in their 20s and 30s. That is because they associate being slim and thin , with being physically attractive.

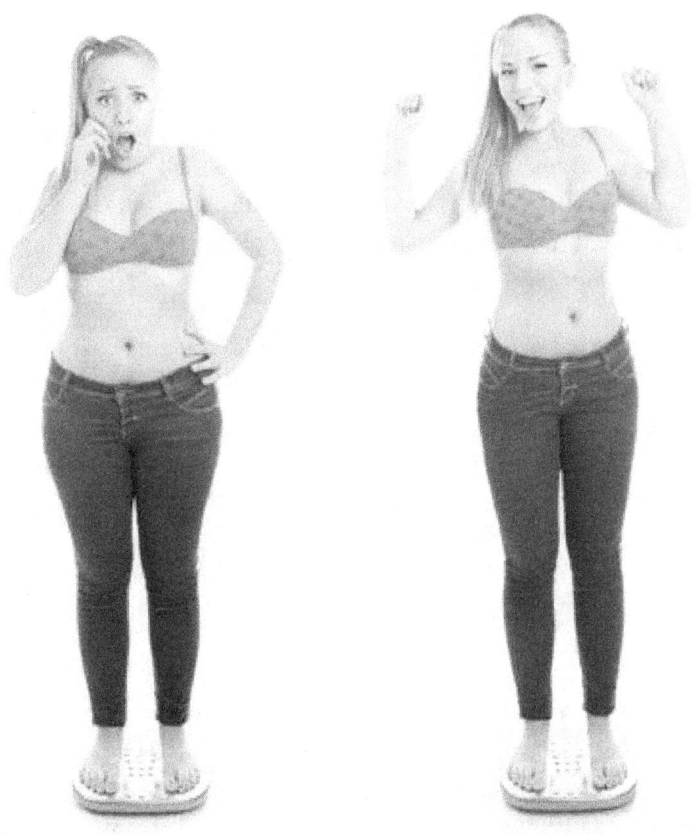

I know drastic dieting is the norm of the day, but you are depriving your body of essential nutrients.

What they do not know is that a human body is going to change as it ages. So your bio physiological and chemical makeup, in your 40s and 50s is definitely going to be different than what it was in your 20s and 30s. So if you think that you are going to be as slim and thin as you were in your 20s, when you are in your 50s, that is not possible unless you have been starving yourself regularly.

Calorie counting can keep you thin. But in order to lose weight or even maintain your weight, you have to keep your calorie intake so low that you are always going to feel hungry. Your body is on starvation mode and demands nutrition. You are not giving it proper nutrition. You are going to be sick continuously because your natural resistance and immunity system is all shot to pieces.

You are not going to have any resistance to disease you are going to take 3 times as long as anyone else to heal, when you are sick and you are always going to feel weak and tired. Do you think this is worth the prospective chance of being ill forever more in order to look as skeletal as Victoria Beckham? I do not think so.

Besides this, you are also going to suffer from low blood sugar or hypoglycemia, because you are always been to be walking around hungry. Do not blame me if one fine day, you collapse, and have to be hospitalized because you are suffering from malnutrition and the accompanying diseases brought about through this slow starvation.

Also remember that the damage done during the starvation years are never quite going to go away. You are always going to suffer from ill health, in the future.

Why are so many famous stars hiding signs of ill health, brought on by starvation? That is because their managers did not bother to tell them that all those diets were doing harm to their bodies. All those tantrums and prima Donna acts thrown by stars can be avoided if they are caught by the scruff of their necks and fed good healthy, nutritious meals.

That is because low blood sugar means low energy levels. It also means bad temper, loss of concentration, and a muzzy outlook towards the world and your surroundings.

If you strictly restrict calories throughout your life, you are not going to get enough nutrition to keep you healthy. So for all those people counting calories, stop doing that, if you are basically a healthy person. It is only when your doctor asks you to watch your calories because you are suffering from some ailment and a restricted diet is heal your problem, that you need to follow his advice.

Diet pills Fads

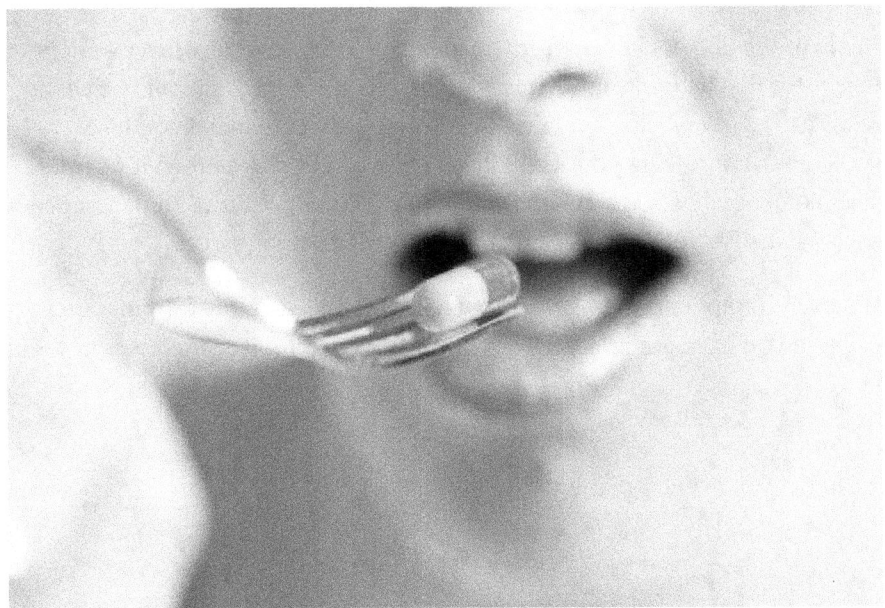

Are you using these pills as a nutritional supplement in place of natural, healthy food, or have you got on to the diet pill bandwagon?

Did you know that the diet pill industry all over the world is more than 120 billion dollars? That is because excessive and extensive marketing has made a large majority of people believe that diet pills are going to solve our weight problems. This is misleading and this is not true.

There can be any number of reasons for your weight problems. You may genetically be inclined to fat. So eating diet pills means that you are not providing your body with the essential nutrients it needs to keep functioning naturally and properly.

But the moment you go to a doctor, and tell them that you have a weight problem, he is immediately going to give you the latest diet pills, given to him by a sales man handing out free samples. He is not bothered much about the state of your health, because the moment you start starving, and suffer from diseases caused through malnutrition, you are going to going to come to him for proper advice.

And then he is going to hand you a prescription for expensive medicines, especially those made up of nutritional supplements.

Many of the doctors have already made up their minds that when a patient tells them that he has trouble staying thin, that he is a glutton, and he cannot resist eating too much. Actually diet pills are meant to make you lose weight by suppressing your appetite so that you cut down on your calories. The moment you stop taking these diet pills, your appetite is going to come back again. So you take more diet pills in order to repress it.

Believe it or not, these pills are about as dangerous as habit-forming drugs because you have got hooked on them. Your doctor did not tell you that, did he?

Quick Weight Loss Diets

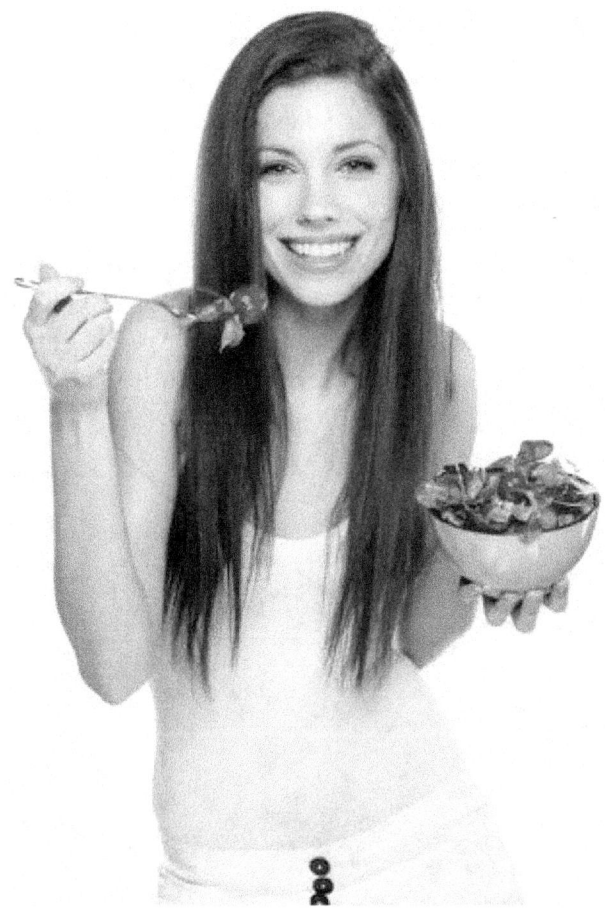

There are so many quick weight-loss diets being advertised in the market today, that many people do not know that most of them are not potentially dangerous, but they are also fads. All you need to have is an important start endorsing them. You go on to these quick loss diets, and you are very glad that you have lost weight.

And then when you stop the diet, there is the weight being added to your bulk again.

Remember that these quick weight loss diets may cause a temporary loss of weight, but they are definitely going to be harmful in the long run because they are teaching you bad eating habits.

Do not go in for drastic diets endorsed by film stars. These diets are going to harm your body physically and it is going to take anywhere between 2 to 3 years for you to get back to your normal state of good health. Long diet routines and plans are also a no-no.

Believe it or not, there is going to be a long-term detrimental physical, and mental effect any sort of starvation diet on your body. I would not be surprised that Beyoncé, who was advocating a large number of detoxification diets around 2008 has not begun showing the bad effects of this starvation Regime, through health problems now and in the future.

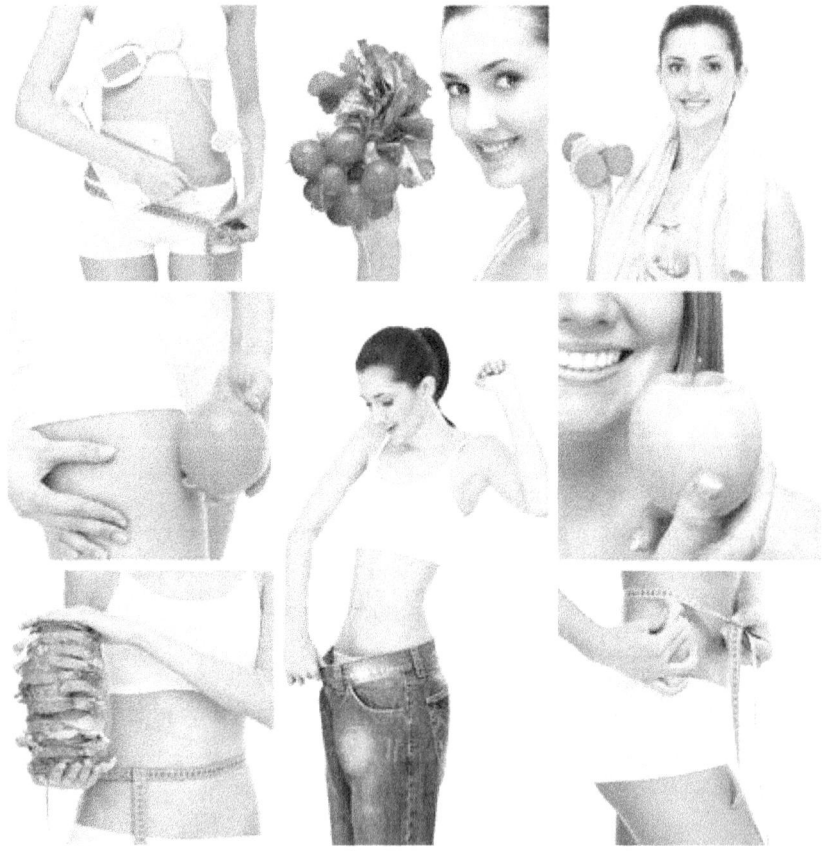

Note that any sort of dieting is a psychological shock to your body system. It considers itself to be in emergency mode because it is not getting suitable nutrients and less food, because you have decided to starve it.

Instead, try the sensible way in which you can lose weight fast and consistently. Start eating 4 times a day. Yes, it is true; when the body starts getting regular meals, 4 times a day, even if they are in very small portions, it starts adjusting itself to this sort of eating routine. Interrupted meals and meals missed are definitely not helpful ways in which you can lose weight. The body just starts accumulating fat, because it does not know when it will have to fall back on that fat as an energy source.

According to the experts on http://www.momswhothink.com/lose-weight-fast/how-to-lose-weight-fast.html, you need to consult a doctor before you go in for any sort of diet program. That is very sensible, because the doctor is going to tell you whether you can afford to starve your body for even a couple of days.

Personally, sensible diet experts like me are against drastic dieting, because I know that that weight is going to come back again, once you have gone back to your regular diet.

Also, let me repeat a story about how I went on a diet, just once in my life and why I say no dieting ever!

So here I was getting ready for a special occasion, which had to take place in a week's time. And I intended to lose about 4 kg. So I took the advice of an Israeli professional army officer friend of mine who told me about the Israeli army diet, where those healthy soldiers keep their weights at a steady 72 kg through a drastic six-day diet.

First two days-absolutely nothing but apples.

Next two days – chicken, chicken, and nothing but chicken

The last two days – cheese, cheese, and just cheese.

Liquid intake – fresh fruit juices.

They lose up to five kgs with this drastic diet. Did you notice that there are no green vegetables, no cereals and many other items from different food groups, not present here.

Well, I am different genetically and I lost 4 kg in six days of drastic dieting. But the repercussions were that I took about three months to get my temper and normally calm and peaceful state of mind back, because I had starved for six days.

And starvation is not conducive to a happy state of mind, especially because I had been starving myself of essential nutrients . It took me 1 ½ years to get my state of good health back because of those days of not eating healthy nutritious food.

Naturally, that weight came back on within a couple of months. Along with accompanying and expected backlash for that starvation which took my system about 1 ½ years to get regulated back to my natural healthy state of physical well-being.

So never try any drastic diet, just because somebody recommended it. Those army officers work out doors training for about 6 to 8 hours every day, I think. I spent those days, sitting in front of a computer. I hardly ever exercise. So I may lose weight temporarily, but never permanently.

Nevertheless, a proper way of getting rid of some of those extra kilos can be done by regulating your meals and adding these items to them – plenty of fresh fruit and vegetables, fresh fruit juice, lean meat and fish, cereals, low fat dairy products, beans and lentils. This diet does not necessarily mean a boring meal routine.

Pep them up with spices like rosemary, thyme, sage, garlic powder, onion powder, and chilli powder. Add a pinch of salt and pepper, and there you are, you have tasty and healthy items which are not only a good way for you to lose weight, but also just about the best way for dieters to lose weight fast!

Try adding more flavor to your food by buying herbs which you can plant in pots on your kitchen windowsill. You are going to get a regular source of fresh herbs. If you do not have a green grocer near you or a good fruit and vegetable store that sells fresh herbs, get this herb garden on your window.

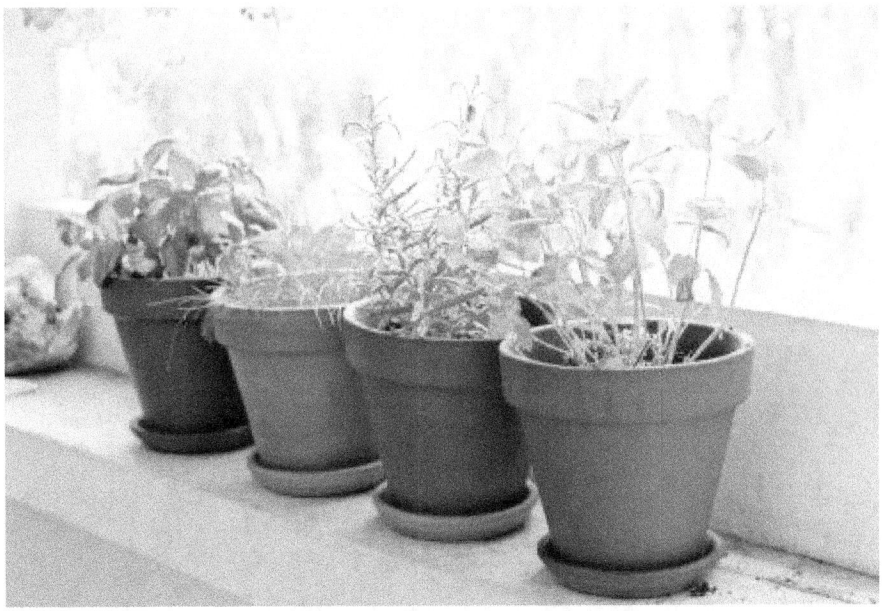

These herbs grow equally well under lights. As long as they are watered well, you can even grow them on a bookshelf, if you do not have a windowsill!

You can start your kitchen garden with rosemary, basil, chervil, chives, tarragon, mint and thyme. Just picking up the herbs and adding them to your dishes are going to make all the difference between a bland, boring dish and something tasty.

Weight Watchers Diets

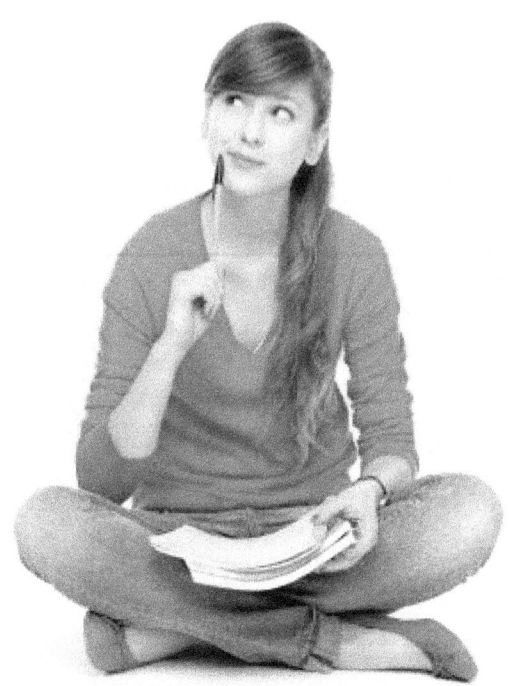

How many calories did I eat for breakfast this morning?

Use this diet only if your doctor says that it is safe for you. He knows the state of your health. The diets are nutritionally sound and do you no harm. On the other hand it may not necessarily do you good, because it does not work for everyone. This is going to depend on your health and your genetic makeup.

So, which is the best diet imaginable, which allows you to eat everything you want, and lets you lose weight?

Is there any diet out there which allows you to do so? Yes, there is one, which is known as the high-protein, low carbohydrate diet.

High-Protein, Low Carbohydrate Diet

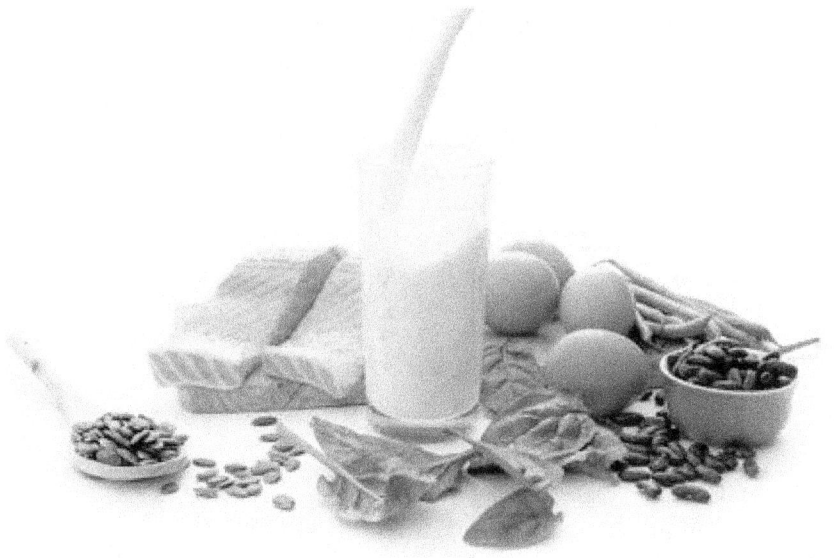

This is among the most popular diets going in the Weight Watchers world today. The only factor in many variations of the diet has in common is that there is no calorie restriction. However, they are going to restrict carbohydrates.

Carbohydrate foods are those which are going to have a large percentage of sugar. These are going to include candies, soft drinks, and cakes. You are also not going to eat any starch -based foods like breads, cereals, pasta, potatoes and corn.

Instead, you can eat poultry, fish, meat, butter, eggs, oil and margarine to your heart's content. These do not have any carbohydrates.

Many people are going to say that this diet is very high in saturated fats. But understand that you are not going to be gorging exclusively on butter and cream. You are going to be eating eggs, and beef, and other items.

Also, everyone is going to get sick of eating roast beef, steaks, very rich food every day, will not you?

So you are going to find yourself eating all these food items in reasonable quantities. Also, the idea that your diet has to be completely fat-free is very dangerous. Your body needs a large amount of fat in order to keep functioning properly. So if you stop eating butter, cream cheese, sweet or sour cream, beef, lamb, liver, and shrimp because you think it very rich, you do not have to make do with other bland and boring items.

Instead, you can vary your diet with soy flour, skim milk, and veal. If you have been programmed since childhood to say no to butter, thanks to the dietary preferences of your parents, try olive oil instead.

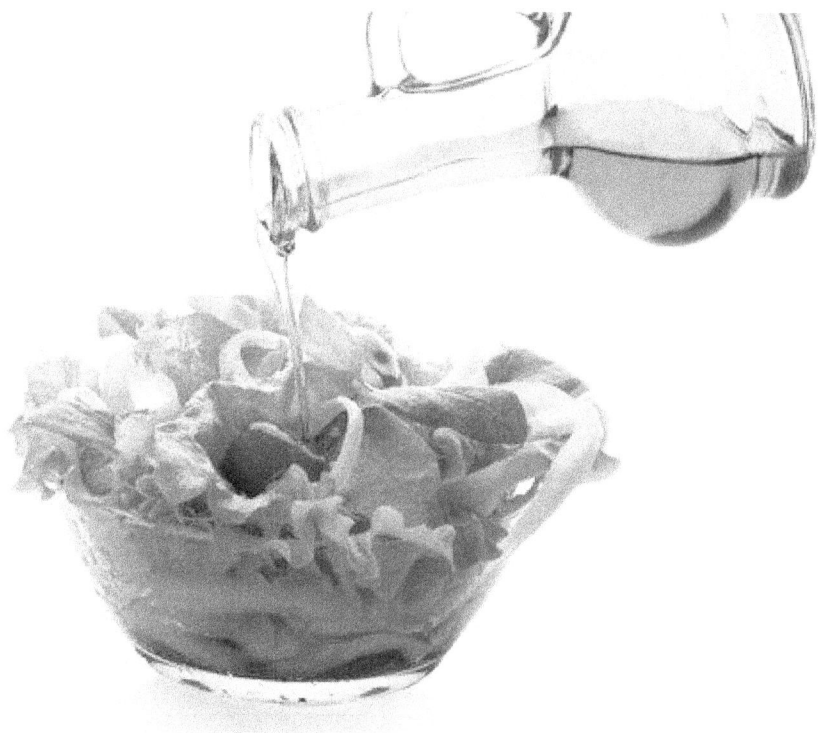

Do not starve yourself, by not eating foods which somebody has told you is not good for you. Believe it or not, the Americans since 1930, decided that butter was fattening, and so was cream, because some doctor had told them so. These were made up of unhealthy fat. And that is why they began on zero fat diets.

And soon they began to stop eating foods which had fat. They also began trying out diets, especially detoxification diets, which made them drink a terrible food combination of maple syrup and cayenne pepper. Believe it or not, they believe that this was the best way in which they could detoxify their bodies. This was in the 40s.

Do you see any healthy nutritional constituents in maple syrup and cayenne? What do you think is going to happen to a system which has been drinking this continuously for 20 days or more?

So remember, if you are suffering from hypoglycemia – low blood sugar – just because you have stopped eating proper meals or are skipping them, there is the chance that you are going to suffer from diabetes later on in your life.

Make sure that you look for a diet, which suits you the best, and then discuss it with your doctor. He will know you and your blood chemistry. Once you have made the choice, make sure that you are monitored occasionally by your doctor, just in case you have lost more weight than is good for you.

Low carbohydrate Diet Tips

Even though I am not a tea and coffee drinker, I would suggest experimenting with different coffee blends, especially if you are a confirmed chocoholic. Some chocolate and coffee blends are quite tasty. In the same way, you can also experiment with tea blends. Some flavors do not need any sweetening at all, including fruit flavors.

Low-carb fruits include melons, peaches, berries, apricots and tangerines. Low carbohydrate vegetables include cauliflower, spinach, mushrooms, green beans, asparagus, cucumber, peppers, and zucchini. These were the tables are also very low in calories. They are also a rich source of minerals and vitamins. High carbohydrate vegetables are lima beans, corn, beetroot, fees, and sweet and white potatoes.

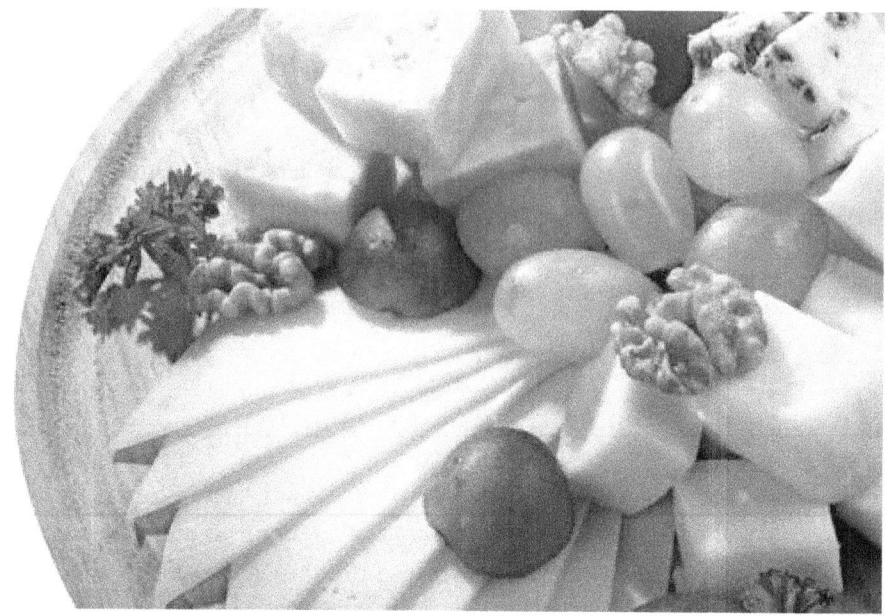

A large number of processed foods, including meat have corn syrup added to them in order to preserve them. Consider this one of the most dangerous things, which has been used for a long time by manufacturers, in order to process food items and to keep them for a long time.

Instead of using cereals for flour, use soy flour. This is excellent for baking, especially when you are making bread. Flour bread, made up of wheat is going to be very high in carbohydrates. Soy flour has more proteins and a lower carbohydrate content.

A number of the salad dressings, which are available in the market nowadays, including mayonnaise, even if they are low-calorie ones – are very high in carbohydrates. So if you are looking for excellent salad dressings, try making your own combination of balsamic vinegar, little bit of garlic, olive oil, and fresh lemon juice. Use 2 – 3 parts of oil to one part vinegar or lemon juice

Best Low Carbohydrate Food Items

There are a large number of food items, which are extremely useful ingredients, especially when you are using them for low carbohydrate cooking. Many of these may have disappeared from your menu altogether, because you have been so influenced with an overload of information dinned into you, that they are not good for health or they make you fat.

That is why you are missing out on some of the most delicious as well as nutritious of food items available to you out there.

Here are some of these food items listed below, which you can use extensively in your recipes and not bother about carbohydrates.

Cheeses

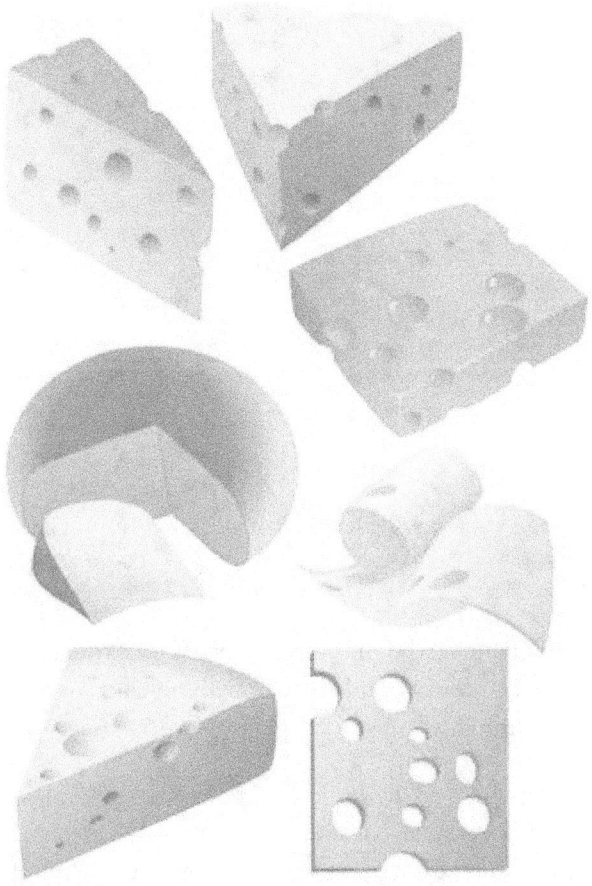

The most popular cheeses which add zest to your cooking are Swiss Gruyere cheese, Parmesan cheese and Ricotta. Farmer's cheese is an excellent cottage cheese and ricotta is the Italian form of cottage cheese. Ricotta is smooth and delicious, and that is why you can use it as a filling for cream rolls and cakes.

Ricotta cheeses are normally unsalted. The Italians use them for cheesecakes and pastries such as cannoli. They also make ice creams with ricotta! That is because this is excellent for absorbing different flavors.

Tofu

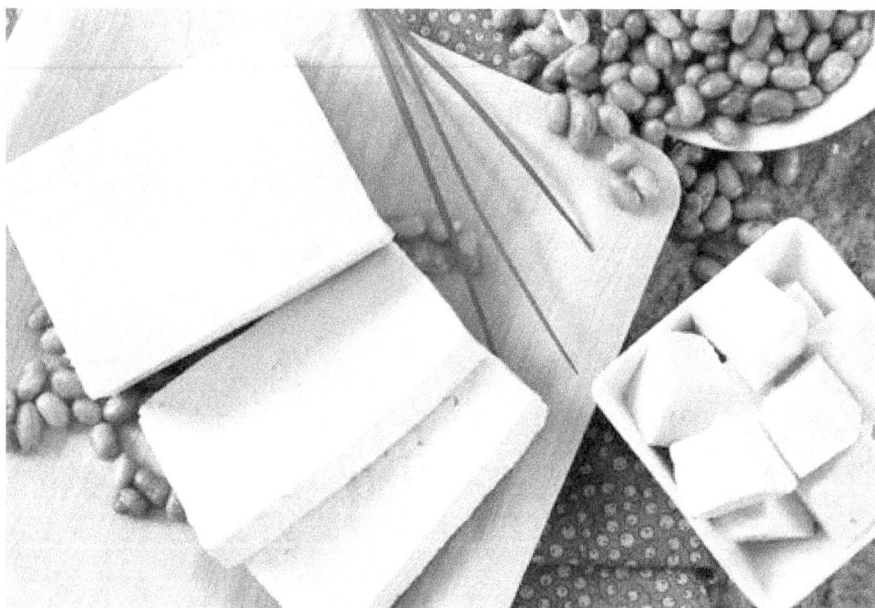

Be grateful to the person who introduced Tofu to the Western world. Until the middle of the 18th century, this was something eaten mainly in Japan and the areas surrounding it.

 These little cakes of bean curd are made from soybeans, and they are an extremely good and inexpensive source of protein. They absorb the flavors of the dishes in which they are port valve and are particularly suited to the taste of soybean sauce. Tofu is used extensively to make sukiyaki. You can also cut them up into cubes, dip them in soybean sauce and use them as appetizers.

Healthy spice powder

This is originally a Chinese 5 spice powder, made up of Chinese herbs and is found in speciality shops. But I made it at home with equal parts of powdered cloves, powdered cinnamon, thyme, star anise, peppercorns, and powdered aniseed. Just try it sprinkled on roasted pork. I did not have Chinese Schezuan peppercorns, so I had to make do with ordinary fresh peppercorns.

Bok Choy

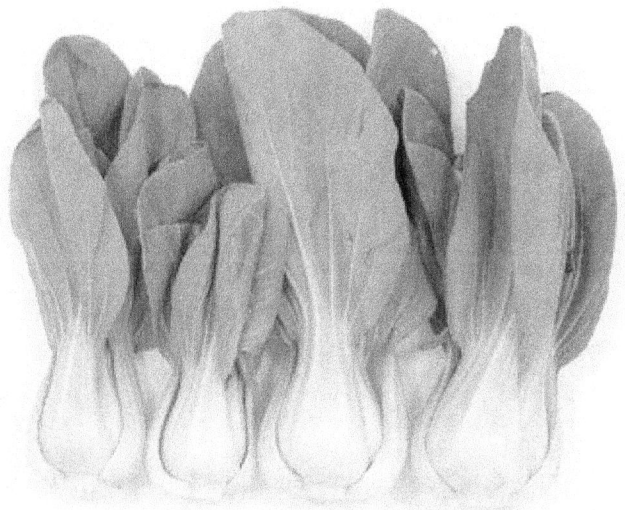

This is also known as Chinese cabbage. You can consider it to be across between cabbage and celery. Use it as a stirfry vegetable or in salads.

Soybean Sauce

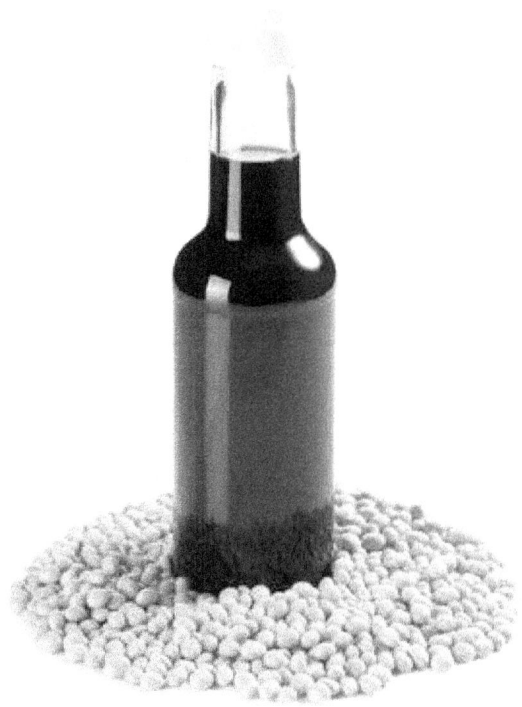

The difference between the soybean sauce you get in the Western markets and the original Chinese soybean sauce is about as much as salt water and distilled water. That is why if you can get original soybean sauce from any Chinese specialty departmental store, buy it. You get it from mainland China, along with Japanese Kikkoman soy sauce. Also invest in some Kikkoman rice vinegar.

These items have very low sodium content, when compared to their American branded counterparts. So what would you like?

Eggs

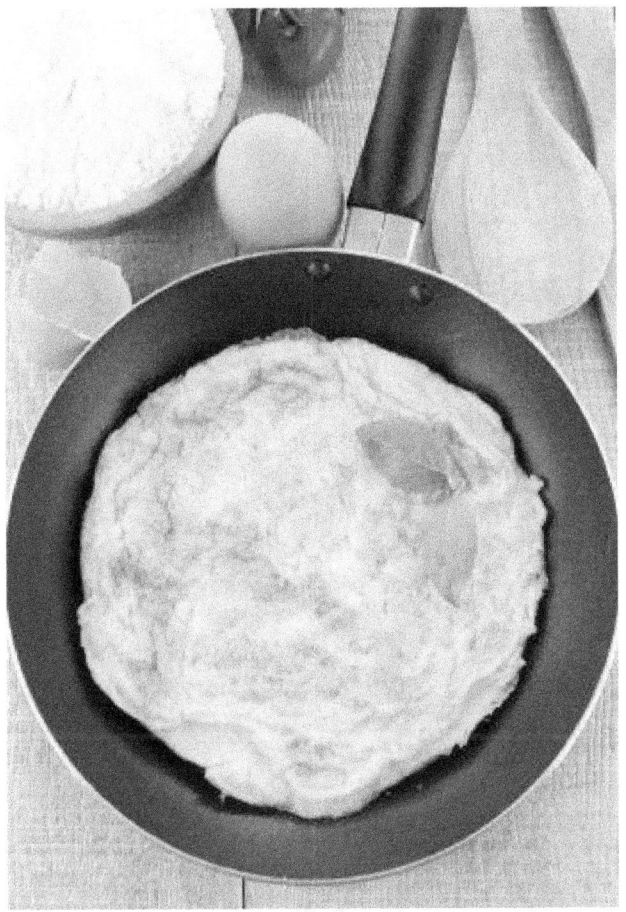

These are of course one of the best buys in protein. Buy them fresh, as far as possible. You can test how fresh and Agatha by immersing it in cold water. If it lies flat, it is fresh. If it sits up, it is not fresh. If it bobs up to the surface discard it immediately!

If you are using egg for baking and have stored them in your refrigerator, then bring them to room temperature, by immersing them in warm water for 5 to 10 minutes.

Mayonnaise

The mayonnaise you get in the market today has plenty of sugar, so it is best to make your own.

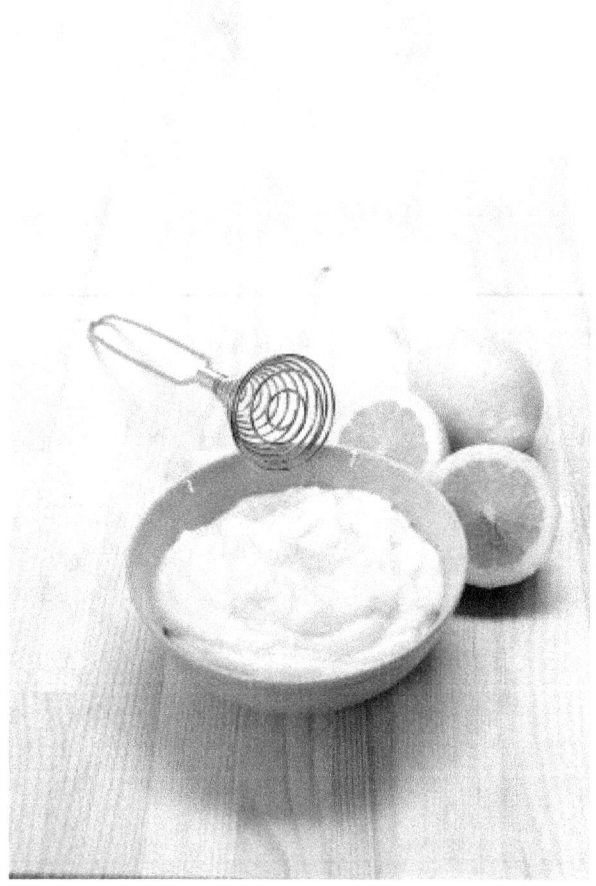

In America, mayonnaise is considered to be a salad dressing. It is actually a sauce.

Aioli sauce, the traditional Italian garlic sauce, is just mayonnaise, with plenty of herbs and garlic.

The basic mayonnaise is of course going to be a stable emulsion of egg yolk, oil, vinegar or lemon juice and seasonings.

Olive oil is traditionally used to make this mayonnaise. But many cooks think this flavor to be very strong and that is why they blend it with other oils. Peanut oil, soybean, and safflower oils are good blending oil mixtures.

For the acid content, you can use cider vinegar, tarragon vinegar or white wine vinegar. Lemon juice is used, if you want a white mayonnaise.

Salt is put in just to taste because over salting of this mayonnaise, is going to overpower the flavor and break the emulsion.

Cayenne pepper or paprika is used to give flavor and color to this mayonnaise. You can also add a little bit of sugar, not only to blend the taste of the seasonings, but also to help in the stabilization of the emulsion.

Fresh egg yolks need to be used, because the yolks of stale eggs are not going to give you a stable emulsion. A perfect mayonnaise is going to be shiny, but not showing any visible drops of oil, stiff enough to hold a shape, but delicate in texture, being a smooth emulsion and subtly seasoned.

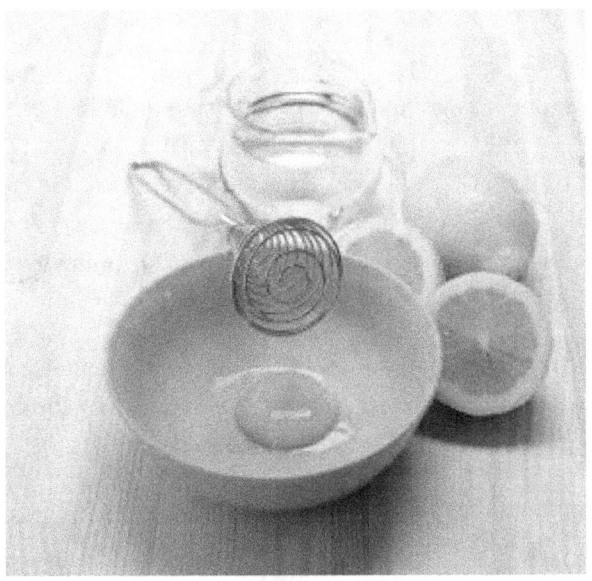

For best results, all the ingredients should be at room temperature. It is a good idea to remove the eggs from the refrigerator at least half-an-hour before use so that they can warm up to the temperature of the oil which has been stored on the shelf.

Blend the dry ingredients, and yolk and a part of the vinegar or lemon juice thoroughly to a paste, before beginning to add the oil.

Add the first few tablespoons of oil drop by drop, carefully so that a good emulsion is formed. Then add the rest of the oil in a stream, beating or whisking constantly.

When the emulsion becomes very thick, more of the ingredients may be beaten in to thin it down, before the rest of the oil is added.

All the oil should be worked in, but it is never wise to try to use more oil than the emulsion will hold. As a rule, the best proportions for a good emulsion to egg yolk to 1 cup of oil and 2 tablespoons whole of vinegar or lemon juice.

It is said, that interrupting the beating process halfway can help in the making of the emulsion, and help strengthen it. However, if you are stopping before the half way mark, start with another fresh egg yolk, beat in the partly made mayonnaise, then continue adding the rest of the ingredients.

Since the mayonnaise is going to thicken on standing, the freshly made product may be a little too thin. This can be finished by adding a tablespoonful of boiling white stock or water beaten in at the end of the preparation. This is going to help in binding the emulsion. Though this is going to thin down the mayonnaise even further, it is going to thicken on standing.

I have noted that happens, when I put the finished mayonnaise in the fridge and leave it overnight. So I have thick mayonnaise ready for next day's breakfast.

However, remember that cold high-temperature going to cause the oil to congeal and separate, so place the bottle in the least corollary off your fridge. Oil is also going to separate, if you have placed it in a really warm place. When this free oil rises to the top, do not try to stir it in because this is only going to increase the separation process.

Instead, remove the excess oil with a spoon or with absorbent paper and use the rest of the mayonnaise as soon as possible.

It may also crack, if you place it on piping hot food! So better keep mayonnaise on the table instead of using it as a garnish.

You can rescue curdled mayonnaise by pulling it together. This is done by starting with one slightly beaten egg yolk then beat in the separated mayonnaise. Add one tablespoonful at a time at first, then gradually increase the amount, treating the curdled mixture as if it were oil.

Similarly, the mayonnaise can be combined by using 1 tablespoon full of water, vinegar or prepared mustard instead of the egg yolk.

In fact, I make sure that my mayonnaise never cracks by putting in one tablespoonful of hot water, and one tablespoonful of prepared mustard, along with other spices right at the very beginning, when I am pouring in the oil in the blender to mix my mayonnaise.

Blender Mayonnaise

The traditional mayonnaise is another tiring to make because you are going to "blend in one table spoon full of vinegar and 2 tablespoons full of oil, and drop by drop, beating constantly; continue beating as the remainder of the oil is added at the spoonful at a time, until the emulsion is thick and then a tablespoon at a time until all the oil is used." It seems our grandmothers had all the time in the world to do that.

I would rather blend this in a ready to mix blender.

For this I need one egg, half a teaspoonful of salt, half a teaspoon of dried mustard, grains of cayenne pepper, 2 tablespoons full of white or plain wine vinegar, 1 cup of salad oil.

Break the egg in the blender container. See, I have not even separated them into yellows and whites. Add seasoning, vinegar and ¼, salad oil. Cover the container and turning water on at low speed. Keep adding the remaining oil in a steady stream, through the cover whole and rest before starting to blend again. Turn off the motor and spoon your thick mayonnaise in a jar. Cover tightly and store in the least cold area of your refrigerator.

This is going to yield 1 1/4 cups.

Chives

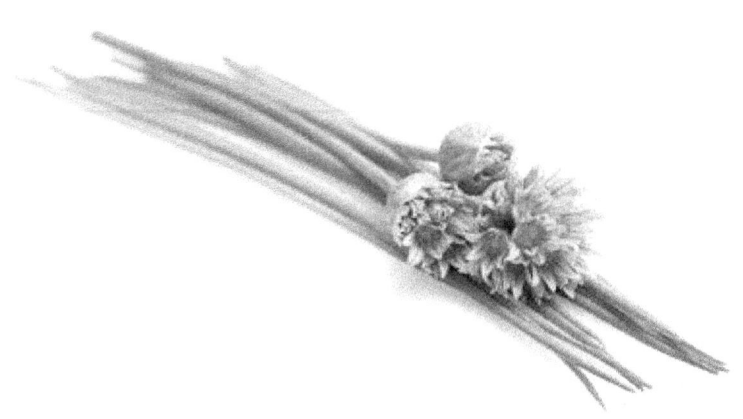

This is an herb which, along with ginger is a delicious addition to eggs, meat, poultry, and cottage cheese. You can buy them either frozen or dried, but fresh are always the best and can be bought at good vegetable and fruit markets.

You can preserve them by chopping them, placing them in an air tight plastic container and then freezing them. You can also grow them on a Sunday windowsill. You do not need to pay much attention to them, because basically chives were considered to be weeds!

Vinegar

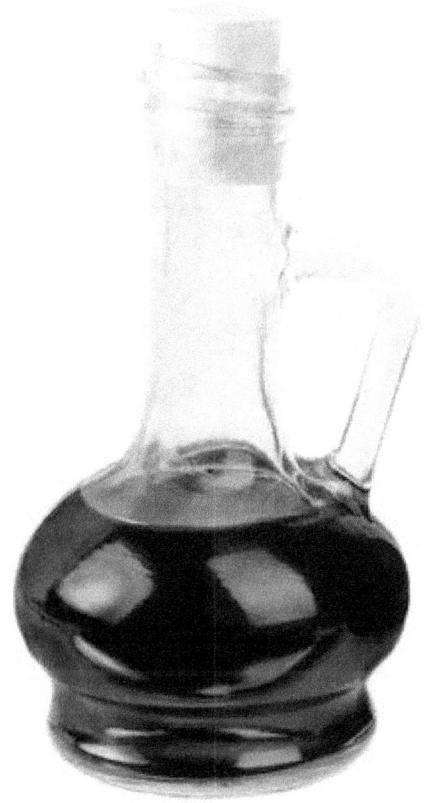

Balsamic vinegar

The best quality vinegar for salads is wine vinegar. You can get plenty of wine vinegar's flavored with tarragon, shallots, lemon, garlic, balsamic vinegar, and even rice vinegar for Japanese and Chinese recipes.

Smoked hams

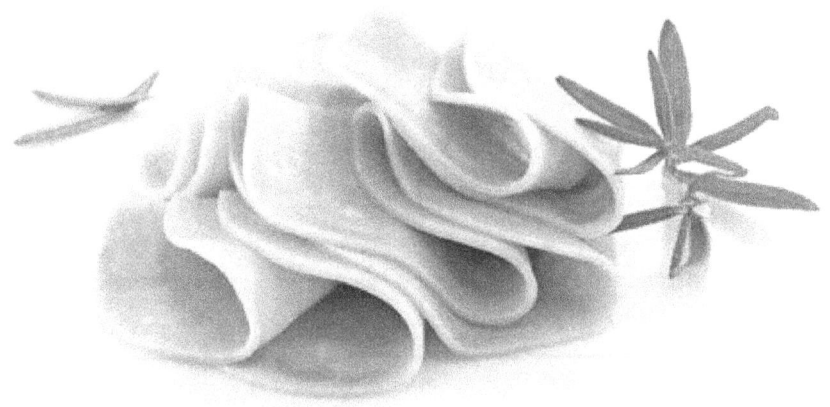

Westphalian and prosciutto should be part of your items list because you can use them as appetizers. After you slice them in thin pieces, you can use your own creativity in making ham salads, ham sandwiches, ham hamburgers or anything else in which you want to add some ham.

Chicken or Beef Stock

If you are making your own stock, that is good. But if you do not have the time, the energy or the inclination to do so, buy canned stock that is because the bouillon cubes or bouillon powder is more concentrated, and that is why the sodium content is going to be more in these cubes. Look for the sodium content in the canned tin. That is why you need make it a habit to read the labels carefully. That is because they are hidden carbohydrates in many foods, which you may have overlooked.

If you have the habit of eating something between meals, boil some chicken or some eggs. You can also cook some lobster, shrimp or crab, if it is easily available. Low-fat cheeses are also good snack items. Just take a couple of bites to take the hungry edge off.

Make sure that you never stuff yourself, when you are at the table. Wait at least for half an hour before you eat anything else. By that time, the blood sugar may have risen so that you do not feel hungry. You feel hungry when you are suffering from low blood sugar, and vice versa. So just take some fruit, vegetables, or boiled chicken and stay the hunger pangs.

Conclusion

All foods are not equal in the decree in which they will make you gain weight, even if they have the same carbohydrate and/or caloric values. If you are fed a diet which is alternatively high in sugar and starch content, the percentage of sugar converted to blood fat is going to be 2 – 5% higher than the percentage of starch converted to blood fat.

This means that any simple carbohydrate food – sugar – is 2 to 5 times as fattening as any complex carbohydrate food – starch –. Therefore, food containing sugar and starch should be kept to a bare minimum.

There are carbohydrate gram and calorie counting sites on the Internet, giving you charts for different foods.

This is an excellent URL

http://www.lowcarbyummies.com/carbohydrate-counter-chart.htm

And so is this.

http://www.carb-counter.net/search.aspx

So, eat healthy, and nutritious food. Look for a diet which suits you best.

Live Long and Prosper!

Authors Bio

Dueep Jyot Singh is a Management and IT Professional who managed to gather Postgraduate qualifications in Management and English and Degrees in Science, French and Education while pursuing different enjoyable career options like being an hospital administrator, IT,SEO and HRD Database Manager/ trainer, movie , radio and TV scriptwriter, theatre artiste and public speaker, lecturer in French, Marketing and Advertising, ex-Editor of Hearts On Fire (now known as Solstice) Books Missouri USA, advice columnist and cartoonist, publisher and Aviation School trainer, ex-moderator on Medico.in, banker, student councilor ,travelogue writer … among other things!

One fine morning, she decided that she had enough of killing herself by Degrees and went back to her first love -- writing. It's more enjoyable! She already has 48 published academic and 14 fiction- in- different- genre books under her belt.

When she is not designing websites or making Graphic design illustrations for clients , she is browsing through old bookshops hunting for treasures, of which she has an enviable collection – including R.L. Stevenson, O.Henry, Dornford Yates, Maurice Walsh, De Maupassant, Victor Hugo, Sapper, C.N. Williamson, "Bartimeus" and the crown of her collection- Dickens "The Old Curiosity Shop," and so on… Just call her "Renaissance Woman") - collecting herbal remedies, acting like Universal Helping Hand/Agony Aunt, or escaping to her dear mountains for a bit of exploring, collecting herbs and plants and trekking.

Check out some of the other JD-Biz Publishing books

Gardening Series on Amazon

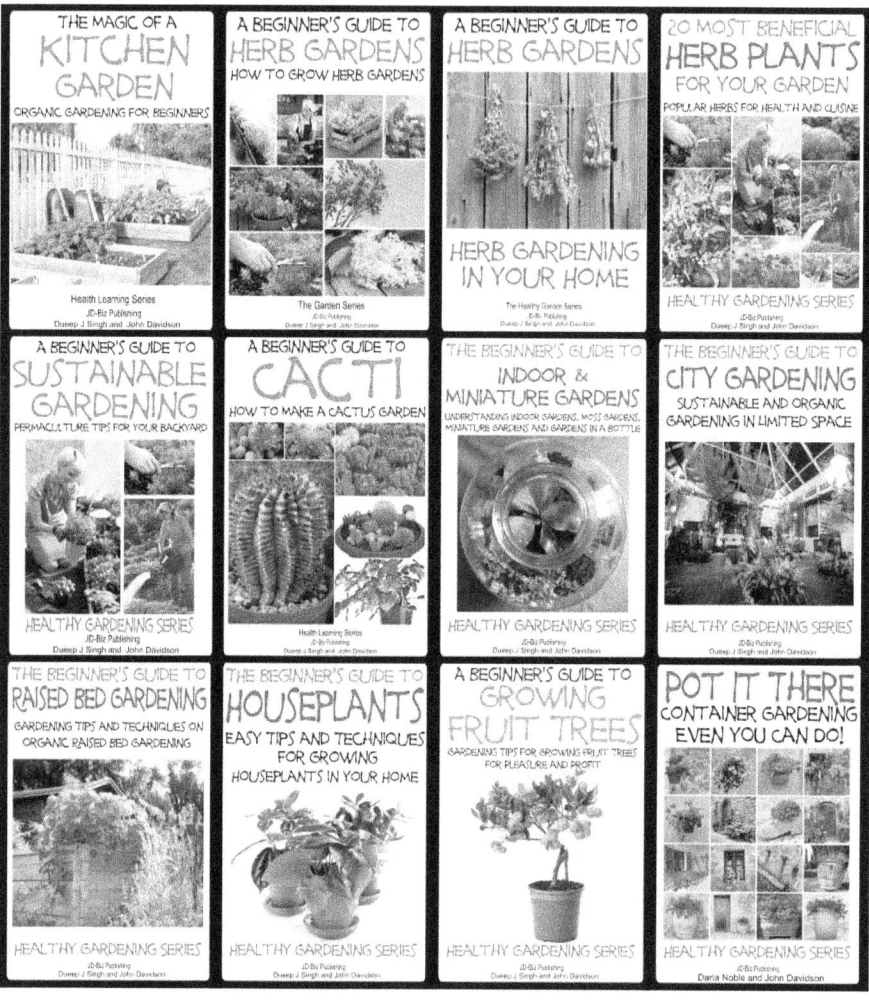

Health Learning Series

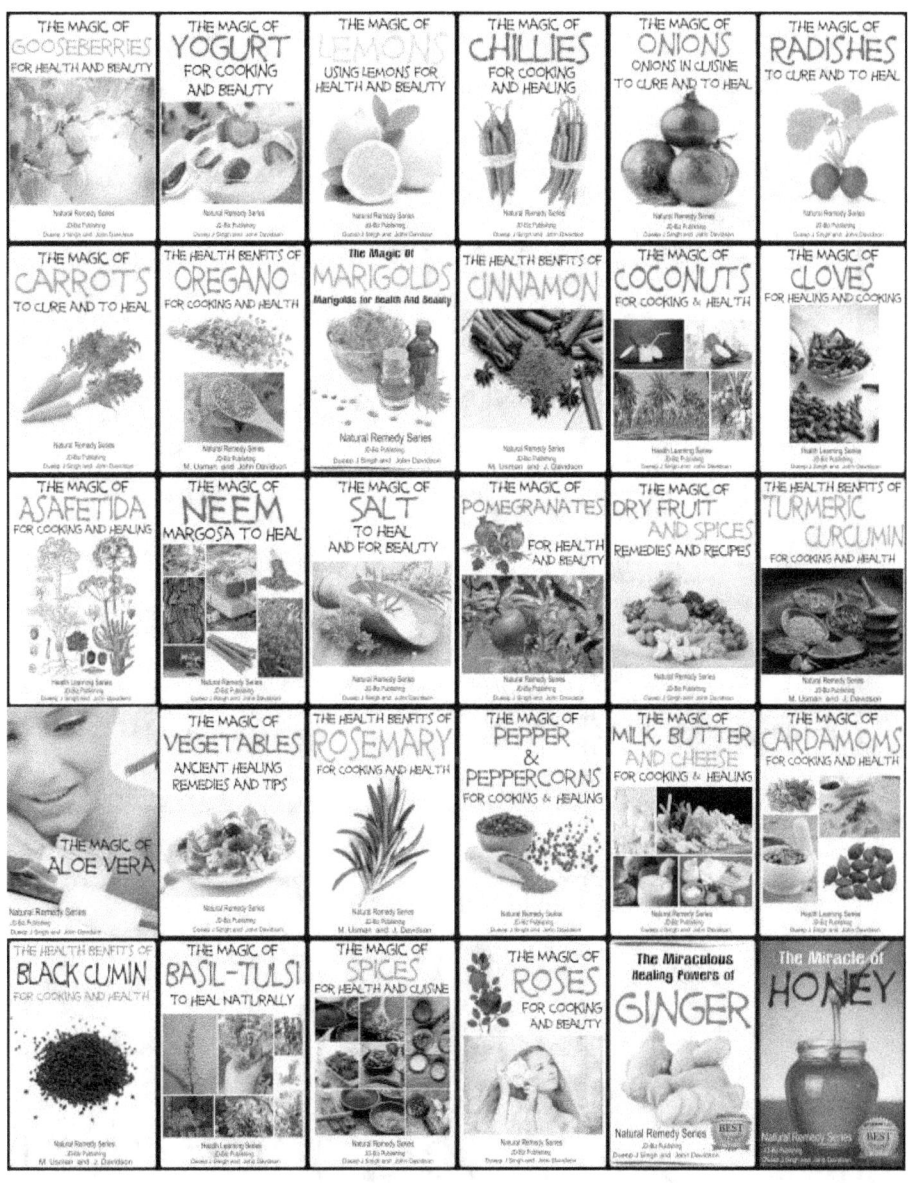

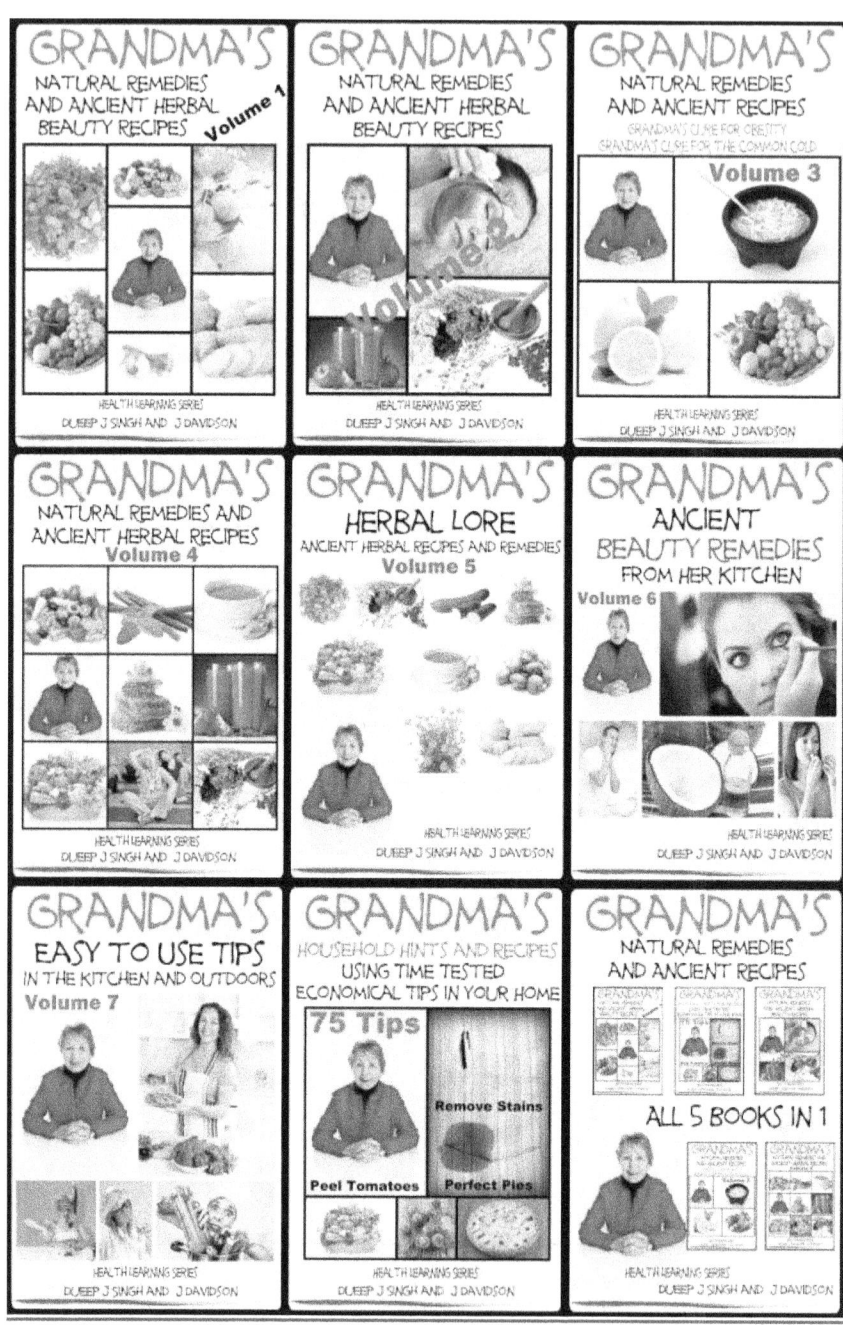

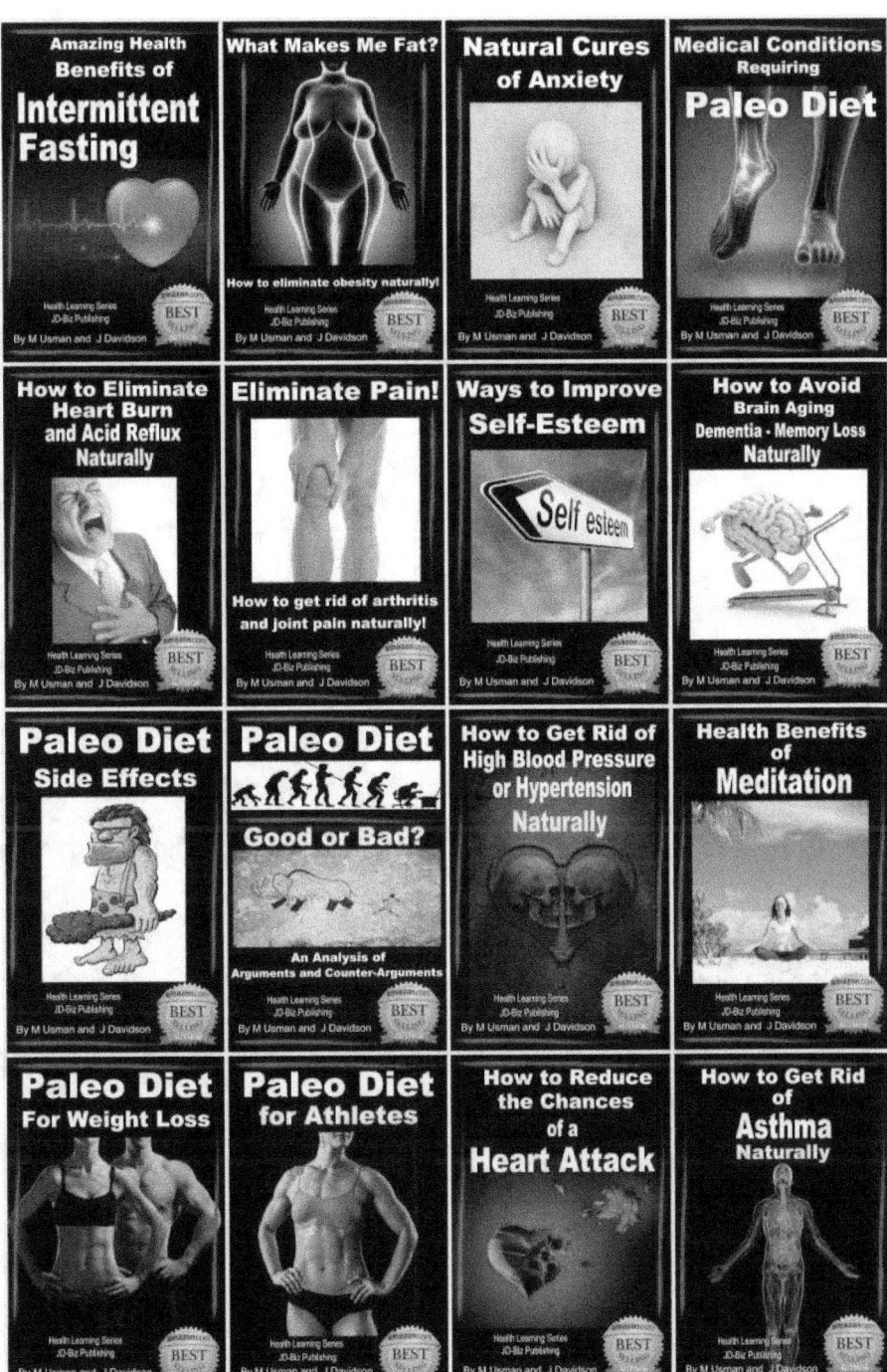

Amazing Animal Book Series

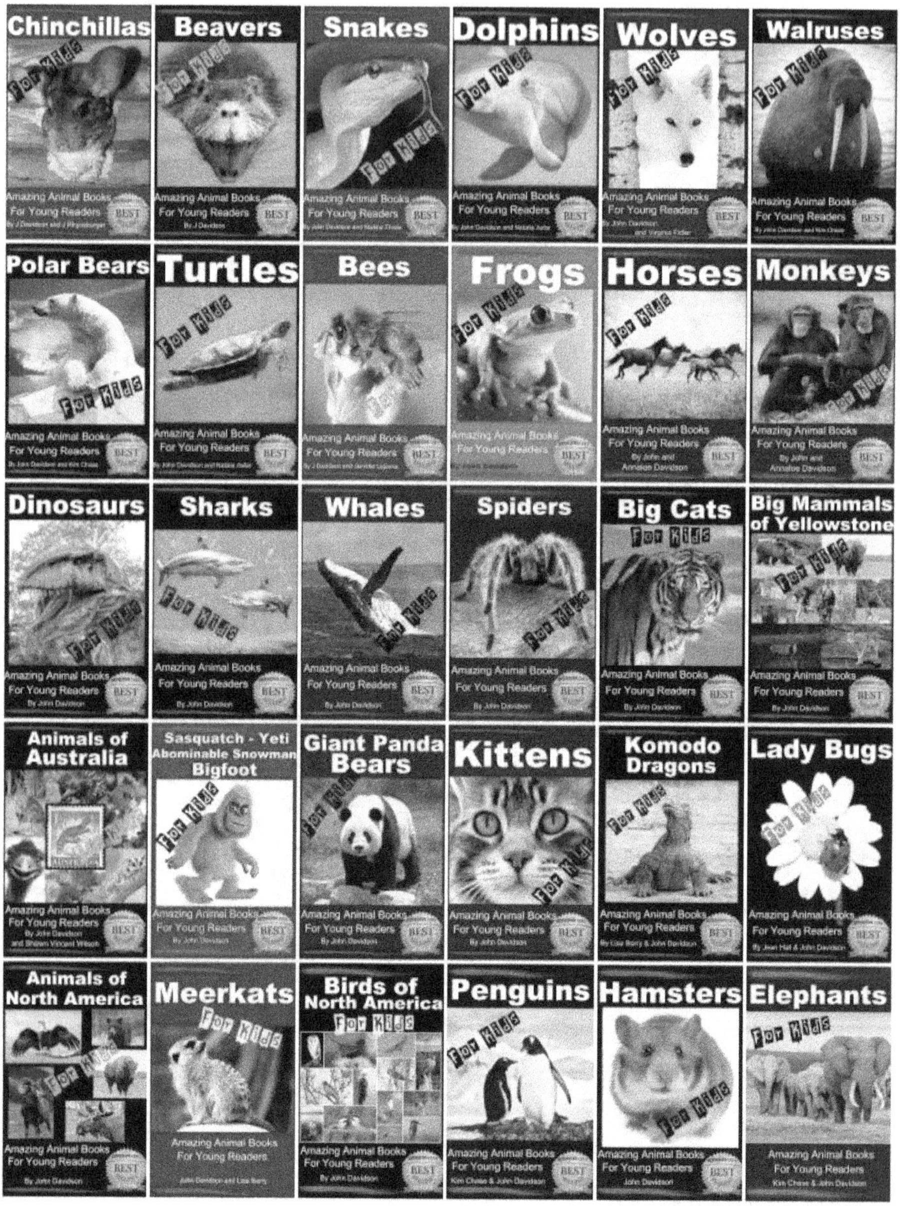

Learn To Draw Series

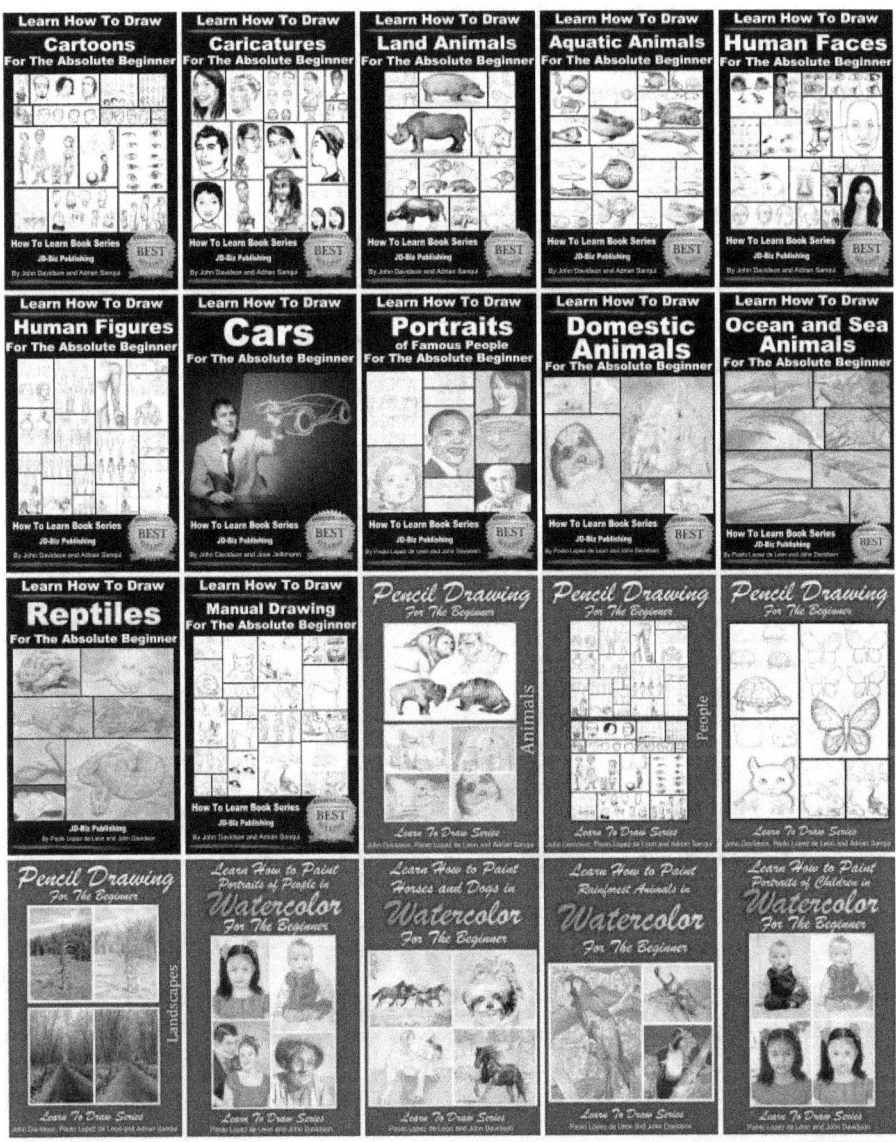

How to Build and Plan Books

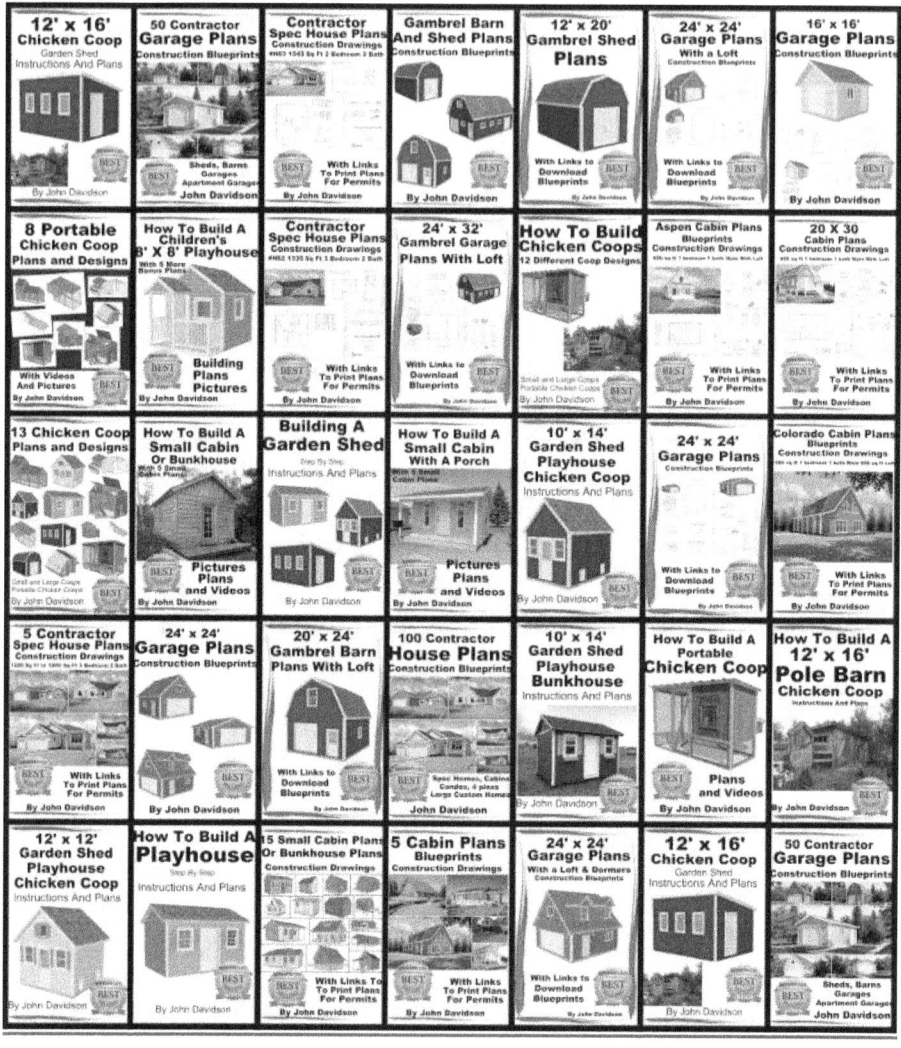

Entrepreneur Book Series

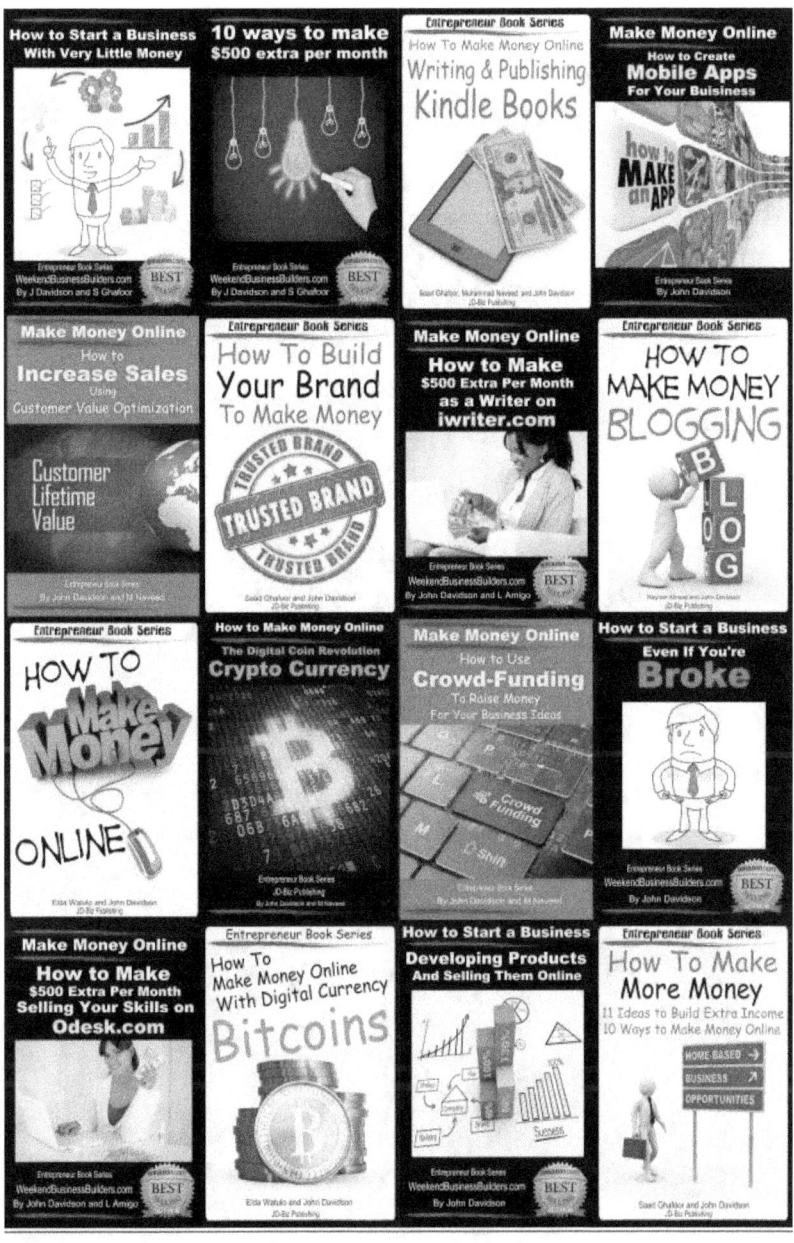

This book is published by

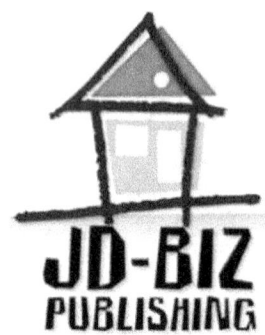

JD-Biz Corp

P O Box 374

Mendon, Utah 84325

http://www.jd-biz.com/

Read more books from John Davidson

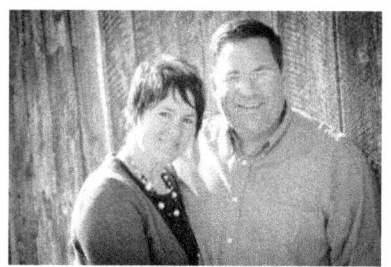

Amazon.com Author Link

Over 300 Books and over 400,000 copies Downloaded

www.ingramcontent.com/pod-product-compliance
Lightning Source LLC
Chambersburg PA
CBHW071135280526
45787CB00003B/1290